QIGONG
THE QUICK & EASY
START-UP GUIDE

by

Frank Blaney

Certified Qigong/Tai Chi Instructor

QIGONG:
THE QUICK & EASY START-UP GUIDE

Less is More Press

First Printing – 2016

ISBN-13:
978-0692655825

ISBN-10:
0692655824

106 1/2 Judge John Aiso Street #707
Los Angeles, CA. 90012

www.downloadqi.com
www.lessismorepress.com

Acknowledgments

This book is "Livicated" to the memory of my older brother who transitioned to the realm of the ancestors and who lived his life with energy and joy;

Patrick Joseph Blaney

&

To my first grandchild who recently joined us in the realm of the living,
& to the courage and fire I see in his eyes;

Elijah Valiente Garvin

Table of Contents

1 – THE QUICK START

You are reading this book because you need something more. You have a health, energy, or life-focus issue that is forcing you to examine, research, and *really* reassess your lifestyle.

We all can learn more about how to enrich this beautiful and brief experience called "life." We all are on a path to learn how to truly live happily, healthy, and with joy for the gift of the life that we experience in each breath.

May this book be a tool and catalyst to make your journey more healthy, enjoyable, and joyful as you seek to achieve your greatest health possible.

We all instinctively know that our **HEALTH** is the foundation of life. Yet we too often treat our health as some sorry joke. Then *something* happens; something breaks, gives out, gets diseased, and all of a sudden you realize you got to change something, and soon.

The "**QIGONG: THE QUICK & EASY_START UP GUIDE**" is written with your situation in mind. Time is short and we really don't have time to weed through a lot of philosophical meanderings and boring scholastic references. It is our health and well-being we are addressing, so let's "keep it real."

We need to make it quick and to the point. This is our health we are talking about. The goal of this easy and quick start-up guide to Qigong is to get you deep breathing, moving, and drinking in the health and well-being that is yours for the taking.

You want to get your life back quick as possible on the fast-track to health?

This book will get you experiencing the power of Qigong in just the few brief minutes it takes you to read it. This really is *THE* **QUICK & EASY START UP GUIDE** to doing Qigong. By reading these brief words and doing the very simple exercises described, you can start feeling the power of Qigong *quickly*, rather than plowing through a lot of reading *about* Qigong. The easiest and most powerful way to learn is to experience something. This start up guide is your tool to experience this fun, easy, and healing gift called "Qigong."

What is Qigong?

Qigong (pronounced "Chi-Gong") is at least 5000 years old. Some people call it "Chinese Yoga." This is not a bad description, since it operates on the same physiological principles as Yoga. What makes Qigong different than Yoga and Tai Chi? I call Yoga and Tai Chi "sisters" to Qigong, but they are very different, just like human sisters can be. Qigong does not involve getting on the ground or getting into difficult body positions, as yoga often does. Qigong involves no complicated footwork or difficult coordination of movements like Tai Chi often does.

Historically, some people believe Yoga came first from India to China, and this "import" was adapted in China as Qigong. My study leads me to believe that Qigong is actually indigenous to ancient China. The roots stem from the Shamanistic practices of rural communities that were the source of ancient philosophical Daoism.

The philosophical concepts within the "Dao de Jing" (400 B.C.E.) have roots that most likely go back 10,000 years to the rural communities along the Yangtze River. The "Yangtze ("Yellow") River was like the "Nile" of ancient China. The Yangtze was where the great and enduring culture of China began eons ago.

Ancient "non-religious" Daoism and Qigong have roots in the same ancient soil; Indigenous Chinese culture, philosophy, and folk healing arts which was where the flower of the ancient Yangtze River civilization blossomed.

So how does Tai Chi fit in?

Tai Chi is a "martialized" version of Qigong designed to incorporate movements from combat and martial arts. Since Qigong is not as complex as Yoga or Tai Chi, it is **much easier** to learn. Yet you still get tremendous health benefits with **a lot less work**.

So why do Qigong instead of Yoga or Tai Chi?

Most yoga sessions last an hour or more. Qigong can be done for just a few minutes a day and still provide profound health benefits for such a small investment of time. Qigong can be done in a very small space (unlike Tai Chi) and requires no special workout clothes or mats (unlike yoga). Many people have experienced injuries doing yoga. In fact, the number one cause of athletic injuries in the United States currently is from Yoga. Americans tend to bring their extreme competitive spirit into Yoga, causing unnecessary effort and strain which leads to injury.

Qigong is so slow and mild, it is almost impossible to overstrain when doing it. The postures and movements are so mild and simple, it is almost impossible to cause an injury. Yoga and Tai Chi are wonderful forms of exercise, but the fact remains; Qigong is much easier to learn, to do, and is safer. *This does not negate the benefits of Qigong's "sisters" as they are truly wonderful mind-body exercise systems.* These factors are simply a reality that may make Qigong a better choice for older, busier, and / or less athletically skilled people.

Most of the movements in this book will take about 5 to 7 minutes to do, including warm-ups! Many people in our fast-paced and modern world feel they do not have time for exercise or mind/body practices. They work many hours to survive in our economically challenging times. They may have people that depend on them like children or elderly family members. They may be experiencing stress from personal, financial, or work problems that would seem to make doing exercises a low priority. This book takes these life realities into account. Reading this book will be easy and doing the movements will be even easier. These are **QUICK & EASY** to do. You will benefit from them.

When I first began Qigong I was experiencing a very difficult period of life. I was working very long hours doing hard physical labor just to survive economically and support my family. I had gone through some very difficult personal challenges and felt threatened from my life's circumstances. I was drinking way too much coffee to keep my "engine running." I was eating unhealthy food. I had gone through a difficult divorce, was tired from the physical labor, worried about my four young children, and my stress made me feel like there was a "knife to my neck" all the time.

I eventually started feeling strong chest pains, getting intense heart palpitations, and I was on anti-depressant medication. A friend of mine who was a PhD medical researcher mentioned that the long term effects of many pharmaceuticals were unknown, since few longitudinal research studies had been done on them. My friend suggested I find a natural and holistic way to deal with my health issues.

I found an esoteric and poorly written books on Qigong at my local library. It took 15 minutes to scan it, noted all the movements that related to my specific symptoms, and I haphazardly strung them together in a 5 minute sequence. I did this for 5 minutes each morning before I sped off to my work site that I had to be to by 7am. Within a week my symptoms were virtually gone and I was able to cease my medication! I felt **significant** relief from just an insignificant 5 minute commitment in less than ideal circumstances. I was hooked on Qigong and eventually took extensive training to become a certified Qigong and Tai Chi instructor.

Congratulations for your commitment to honor your body and mind by learning these movements! It takes significant wisdom and courage to try anything new, especially something "healthy." Simply by regularly doing the movements in this book for just a few minutes a day, you will begin a journey to better health and mental focus. Start where you are at. Do not pressure yourself to be perfect. Make your Qigong time a special renewing experience just for you. It is your gift to yourself.

This book is a *The* **Quick & Easy Start-Up Guide**, so let's start now. After you read this last paragraph, put down the book, close your eyes, and just "**listen**" to your breath for about 30 seconds. Don't try to change it, just notice what it is doing, how it moves, what it feels like and sounds like inside of you. Do that *now*.

2 – EASY PREPARATION

The key to Qigong lies in the breathing. In China, doctors will prescribe a specific Qigong "exercise" to patients who are in hospitals and are bed-ridden. How can you prescribe a Qigong movement to someone who cannot move? Because, *the key of Qigong lies in the deep diaphragmatic breathing and the visualizations that the practitioner imagines in their mind*. That is what moves the "Qi" or bio-electric energy of the body, which in turn, affects the blood flow and circulation, which in turn, delivers oxygen and nutrients to the parts of the body that the mind travels. This point cannot be overemphasized.

Most people begin their Qigong shortly after awakening in the morning. To prepare for

Qigong, get to bed in time the night before so you get enough rest. It is best not to have a full stomach when you do Qigong, so eat something after Qigong movements if you wish,

To prepare for Qigong upon awakening, simply use the bathroom, perhaps take a few drinks of water, and then begin. It is better not to drink stimulants like coffee or tea before doing Qigong. It can disturb the flow of Qi. Drink those kinds of beverages after your practice if you desire.

Begin your practice with some mild stretching that you are familiar with. One good one is to stand upright, interlock your fingers high above your head, stretch your arms as high as possible and press your feet deep into the ground at the same time. Breathe normally. If you are able, turn slightly to the left and right, then slightly to the sides.

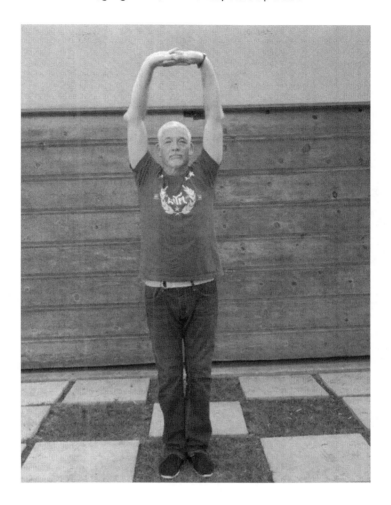

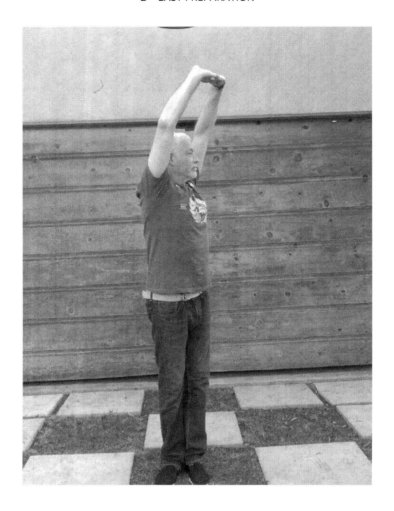

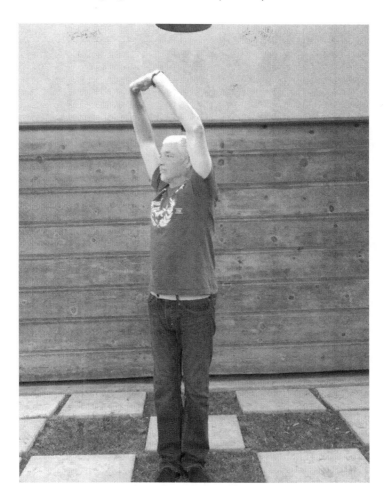

ENTER THIS URL TO WATCH THE DEMO VIDEO:
"Warm Up Stretch"
https://youtu.be/UWqB1dJn4ZM

You can also do simple neck rolls, arm rolls, waist turns, and knee bends. Keep things short, effective, and simple. **Do not force anything or push outside of your range of motion and comfort zone!** To do so is to defy the spirit of Qigong, which is to be natural and relaxed. You

17

are ready and have completed your *easy preparation*. You are ready for Qigong.

3 – EASY POSTURE

Nearly all 10,000 different forms of Qigong start with the same beginning posture or stance. Have your feet slightly wider than shoulder-width apart. Experiment with the placement of your feet until you feel balanced and centered. Asian martial arts and mind-body practices believe the area two inches below our navel in the lower center of our abdomen, to be the center-point of balance and energy. This is where our main "bio-electric battery" exists. We can imagine as we breathe in, that the breath flows into the top of our skull, down our spine, and into this area, called "Dan Tien," in Chinese.

There is a slight bend in the knees at all times. The shoulders are extremely relaxed and soft, and the arms a little away from our torso.

Imagine a "golf-ball" size pocket of air in your armpits between your triceps and torso.

The spine is straight, but not stiff. Imagine a string is attached to the very center of the top of your skull (called the "Bai Wei" meridian point in Traditional Chinese Medicine—"T.C.M.".) The string lifts your skull, which lifts the vertebrae of the neck, which elongates and lengthens the spine.

In your pelvis, imagine you are very slightly tucking your tailbone forward and up just a fraction of a centimeter or so. Tighten the perineum very slightly, like you are trying to prevent urinating. Both of these actions are so mild as to be almost imperceptible. **Do not over think** or over-focus on this too much at the beginning, as it will become second nature over time. The key to Qigong is to *not to try too hard* at anything. Then, things will normally flow easier and more efficiently.

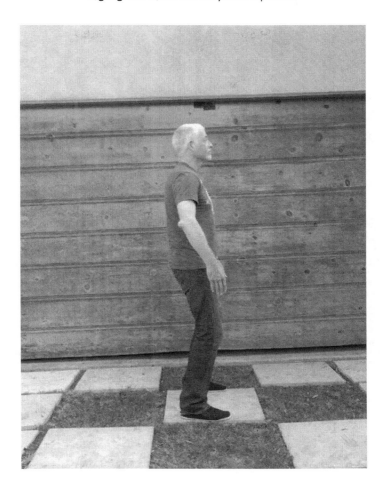

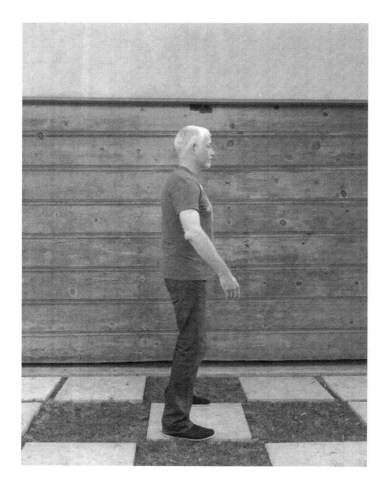

It is usually good to close your eyes and do a brief "head to toe" relaxation before starting the movements. It will relax your muscles, which will allow the Qi to flow more freely. Lightly press the tip of your tongue to the top of the roof of your mouth, just rest it there, do not strain. You can begin to imagine warmth moving from the top of your skull, down your forehead, eye muscles, face muscles, through your jaw, and softening the neck muscles on the way down. Imagine there is warm oil on your shoulders, which is softening them. That warmth and relaxation move down like warm oil dripping over your torso, abdominal muscles, through your pelvis, into your thighs, calves, feet, and into the ground. From the arches of your feet you spring imaginary "roots" that sink 3 feet into the ground. You are centered, relaxed, balanced and rooted.

Now, take just a few moments to simply feel and listen to your breath. Now, you are at peace and ready to drink deep of some power and calm that will ground you for the day ahead. Breathe deep and be thankful to be alive another day.

4 – EASY MENTAL FOCUS

What you just did in the last chapter is the very foundation of all Qigong. All of the 10,000 or more different styles of Qigong around the world, in all of the over 5000 years of practice, rest upon the simple exercise you just did. That is it in the nut shell. Listen to your breath. Breathe deep and diaphragmatically. This is what will increase your awareness of your body, its sensations, needs, signals, and pleasant sensory experiences. Self-awareness and body-awareness is the fruit of regular practice of easy and simple Qigong.

The core of the mental focus within Qigong is traditionally called the "3 Intentful Corrections." I prefer to call them, the "3 Intentful Adjustments," since it is less judgmental in tone and more accurate. These 3 Intentful Adjustments are tools

24

used both by new beginners, and Qigong Masters practicing in the lofty heights of the legendary "Wudang Mountain," the historical and spiritual center of ancient Qigong, Tai Chi, and Kung Fu. Both beginner and master will utilize these same tools, or mental focuses as they do their Qigong movements.

The 3 Intentful Adjustments of Qigong are *Posture, Breathing*, and *Mental Focus.* These three foundations will be periodically "checked in on" with one's conscious mind as you practice your Qigong. The key word is "periodic." **There is no room for obsession with perfection in Qigong**. The quest for so-called "perfection" produces far too much stress. Every now and then as you do the movements, ask yourself questions, like; "*Are my shoulders relaxed?*" "*Am I moving my torso and hips in unison?*" "*Am I breathing deep into my 'Dan Tien*" (lower abdomen area)?" "*Am I calm?*" "*Are my abdominal muscles too tight?*" etc.

Again, these questions are asked just periodically during Qigong practice. I often check on the 3 Intentful Adjustments as I transition from one Qigong movement to another. I take just a few seconds before starting the next movement, and check in to make sure I am in a good posture, my muscles are relaxed, and I am listening to my breath.

The important point to remember about mental focus in Qigong, is where your mind travels, your Qi travels. Some of the more "complex" Qigong forms involve simply standing still and stationary in a Qigong position. The "movement" is actually taking place in the mind, where the mental focus attention is targeted.

I like using this analogy. Doing Qigong is like giving yourself a free acupuncture session. They have identical goals; to move Qi through the body in a balanced manner. In Chinese Acupuncture, they use needles to draw the Qi to specific areas of the body. In Qigong, the "needle" is our mind and its mental focus.

For example, if I am doing a standing Qigong, and I imagine the breath coming into my body being bright, vibrant, red light and I breath it straight into my heart, the Qi flows there, even though my physical body is not moving a centimeter.

If I draw the breath into my abdomen, and imagine the Qi/Oxygen moving in circles clockwise along my large colon, the Qi flows there and assists in my digestion and in the regularity of my system.

If I imagine the Qi coming up from the earth upon which I stand, then flow like a healing river of bright light through my injured right knee, then that is exactly where the Qi flows, just as surely as if a T.C.M. doctor stuck a needle there.

The power of Qigong comes from the connection between the deep diaphragmatic breathing and the mental focus and intention. This is what directs the flow of Qi. The mental focus of Qigong is where the power comes from. We can heal ourselves with this easy and simple ancient mind/body practice.

(For more details, refer to the "3 Intentful Adjustments" in BONUS CHAPTER #14)

5 – EASY LEARNING

Simplicity is a key trait of Qigong. The following set of movements is easy to learn and do. They can be done as a complete set. Each movement can also be done individually as a "stand alone" exercise if your time is short. If you are a bit stressed before a meeting, a challenging conversation, or work task, take just three minutes and do just one of these in an office, parking lot, or even a bathroom stall.

The overall effect of this particular set of exercises is to calm one's spirit and mind. Most Qigong practitioners find it soothing. It is a powerful stress reducer and enhances one's overall mood. Some T.C.M. doctors "prescribe" these movements for mild depression.

As with all Qigong exercises, when you are first learning the movements, you are using your conscious attention in order to remember and perform them. This makes it difficult to get into a *deeply* relaxed state, because your mind is working in a conscious and logical mode. This is normal. Spend your first few moments just consciously "roughing out" the movements, and do not try to get super relaxed or into "the zone." Rather, just take a few moments to feel the movements, remember their basic pattern, and adjust to how it flows. Eventually you will get a basic feel for the pattern and sequence of the movements.

For example, when you are cooking a meal, you do not taste deeply how delicious it is, because you are working at preparing the meal. Once everything is prepared, *then* you can sit, rest, and deeply savor the taste of your delicious meal. Think of learning a new Qigong exercise as "preparing a meal." When you have that down adequately, then you can "taste" the healing relaxation of Qigong movements.

There is an old Chinese saying regarding learning Qigong: "Learn inside, perform outside." It is easier to be undistracted inside, where you are surrounded by the familiar. Learning a new Qigong movement outside forces your limited attention to things like safety of the environment, traffic, etc. But once you are familiar with roughing out the movements, your best option is to do the Qigong outside, so you can get more fresh air into your lungs, more sunlight on your skin, and touch the healing powers of Mother Nature as you do Qigong.

Let's begin with our first easy set of Qigong Movements, "Building the Qi—The Easy 3."

6 – EASY MOVEMENTS: SET 1

("Building the Qi")

This first set of only three movements, is extremely easy to do, and enhances the process of building up our internal Qi. This set is called "Building the Qi—The Easy 3." The movements can be repeated as many times as you desire, and each movement can be done as a separate and self-contained exercise if you have a limited amount of time. The effect of this set is to nurture and build up your own internal Qi, or storehouse of bio-electrical energy. This is an excellent Qigong set for beginners to do as a regular routine.

We start in the beginning Qigong position

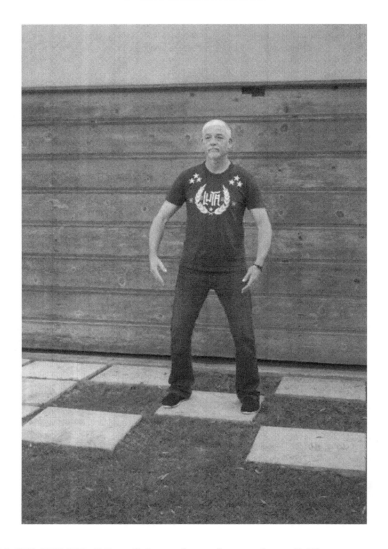

MOVEMENT #1: "Awakening the Qi"

From the starting position, *inhale* as you slowly and gently lift your arms up in front of you to shoulder height. Wrist and hands should be hanging freely from the arms, which should be as relaxed as possible. As you raise your arms you can straighten your legs a little, but do not lose your original posture with the spine straight and pelvis slightly forward. Raise the arms up slowly so that it corresponds to the timing and pattern of your inhalation. As you *exhale*, let the arms down gently in time with your exhalation, stopping just in front of your thighs. The idea is to visualize your movement as gently moving kelp in the ocean or slow moving waves. Let each breath dictate your speed of movement. Think "slow." Do this for as long as you wish or until your arms get tired. IF you feel balanced and want to, you can "rock" forward a bit on the balls of your feet as you lift your arms, then rock back onto your heels a bit when you lower your arms. You can also straighten your legs a bit as you lift your arms, and bend them back down (a bit) as you lower your arms. Experiment! Each body and person is different. Just be sure to stay in your comfort zone.

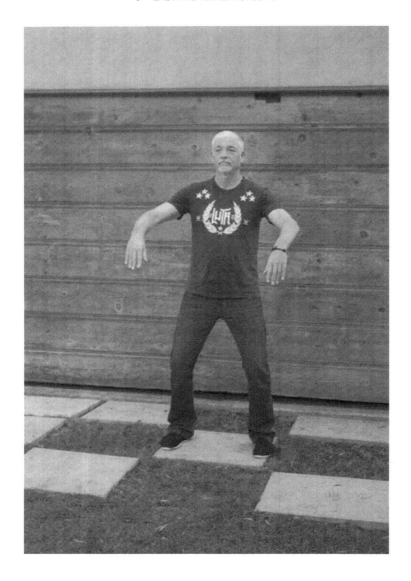

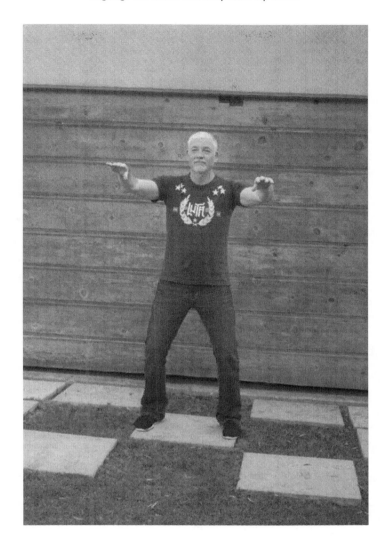

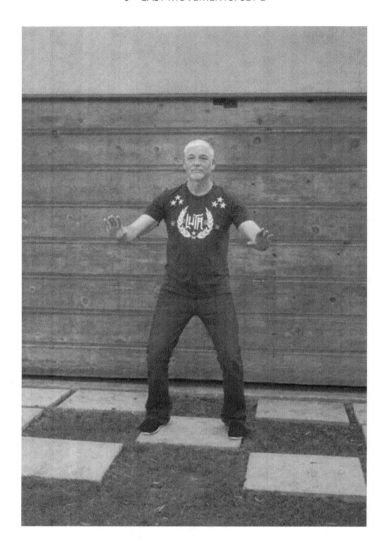

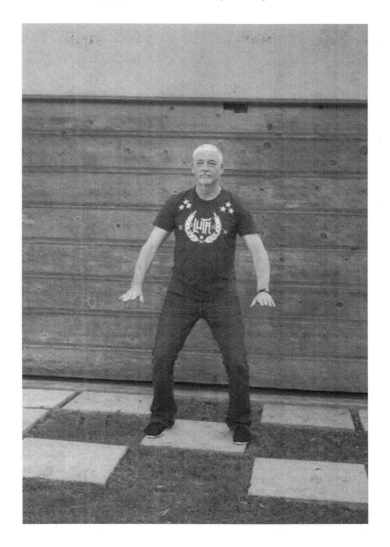

MOVEMENT # 2: "Feeding or Storing the Qi":

After completing the last exercise, let your hands rest at your sides. Let your hands "float" out in front of your belly button, one hand over the other. They should end up about a foot and a half away from your lower abdomen. On an

37

inhale, slowly move your hands towards the area about 2 to 3 inches below your belly button ("*Dan Tien*" in Chinese, and "*Hara*" in Japanese). Continue inhaling as you palms come together in a "prayer" position, moving up the front of your body to about your shoulders or chin while still inhaling. Let your hands and arms separate away from each other and float down as you slowly exhale. Your arm motions will be drawing a semi circle or "orbit" as they move back down towards the original position in front of you belly button. This last movement I like to think of as "the flower opening." This exercise literally stores Qi in its main storehouse of your body, this "*Dan Tien*" area. This exercise is energy building over the long term.

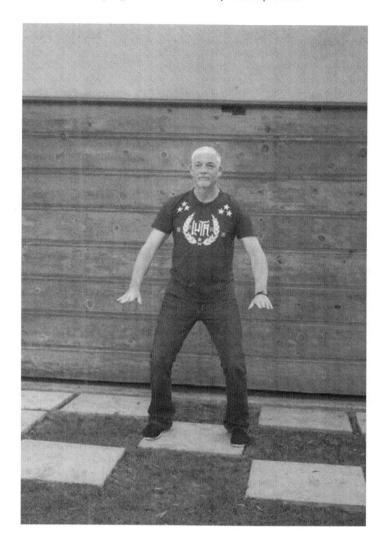

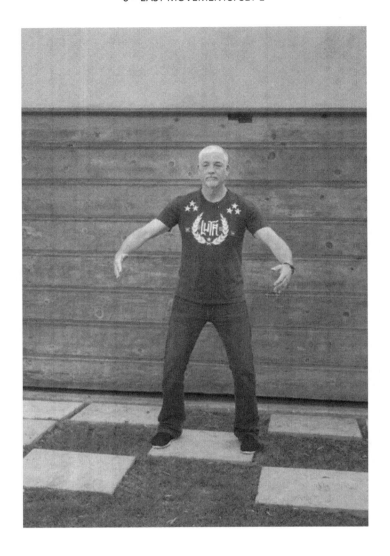

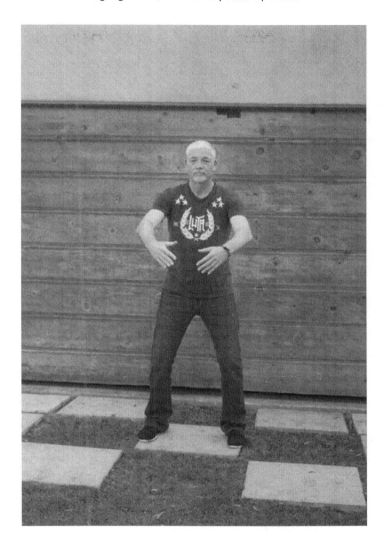

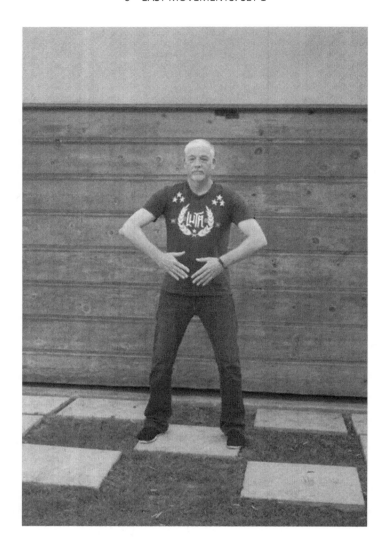

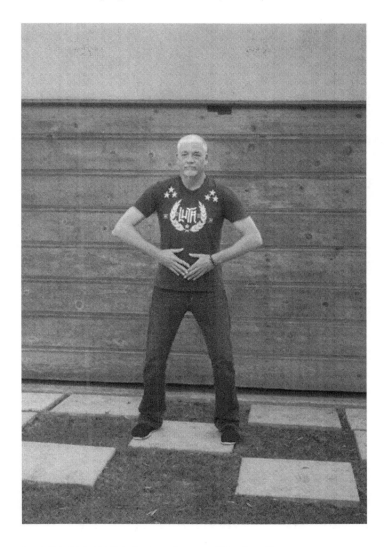

MOVEMENT # 3: "Eagles Flight.":

From the beginning Qigong position inhale as you gently lift your arms from your sides with your palms facing the ground. Let the arms be *slightly* bent as you raise them to shoulder or head level. As you exhale, slowly and gently let them return to your sides. Do not be abrupt or

43

"jerky" with these movements. Visualize an eagle slowly and gently moving its wings. Coordinate movements with the rhythm of your breathing. You can also raise your knees *slightly* as you raise your arms while maintaining the original posture of the spine and pelvic area. Do this movement for a minute or so (not too long or your shoulders may get sore).

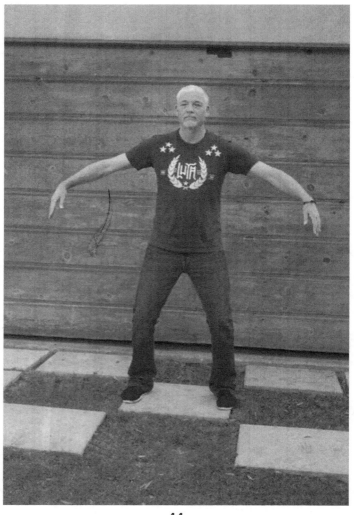

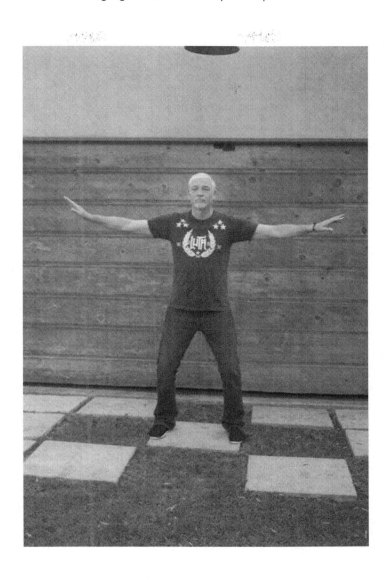

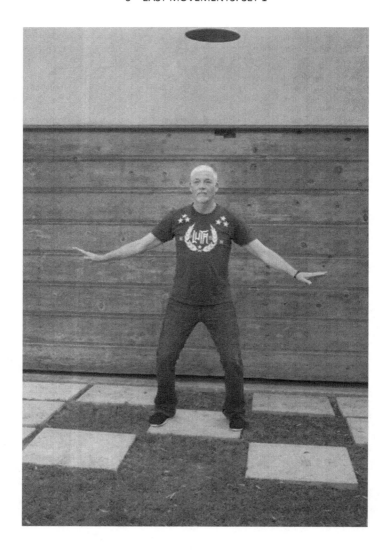

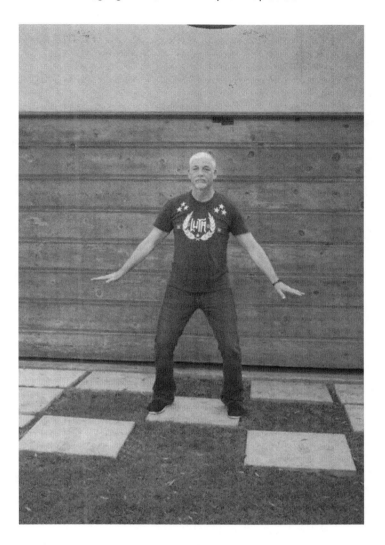

CLOSING: "Sealing the Qi"

Stand in your beginning Qigong position. Open your eyes. Have your arms reach out horizontally from your waist "scooping" in some "Qi/air" towards your lower abdomen. Inhale as you scoop, and exhale as your hands move towards your lower abdomen (in Chinese, the "*Dan Tian*").

47

Imagine you are "pushing" Qi into this area 2 inches or so below your navel. Do this three times. Take at least 30 to 60 seconds, not moving, with eyes open, returning to a normal state of consciousness. Take the time to do this after your Qigong session, so your mind does not feel "spacey" the rest of the morning.

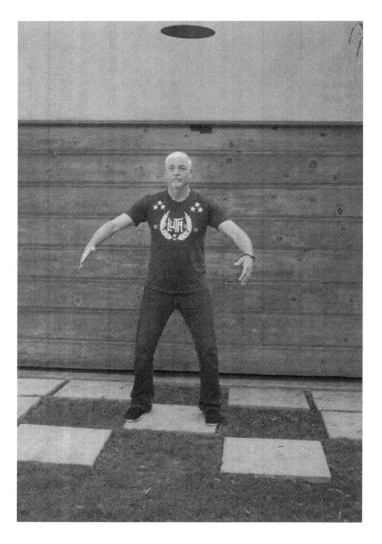

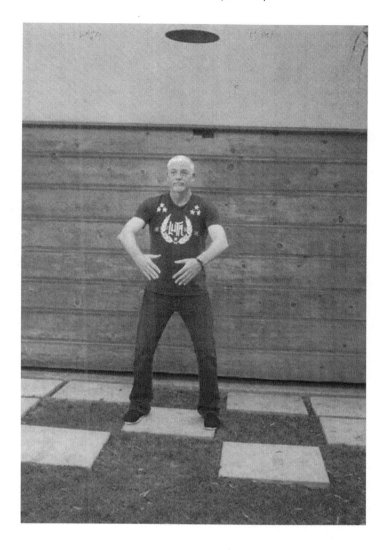

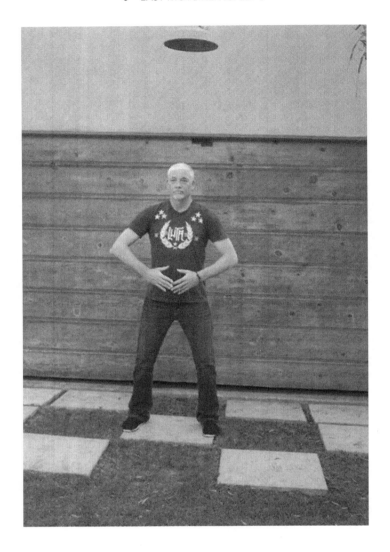

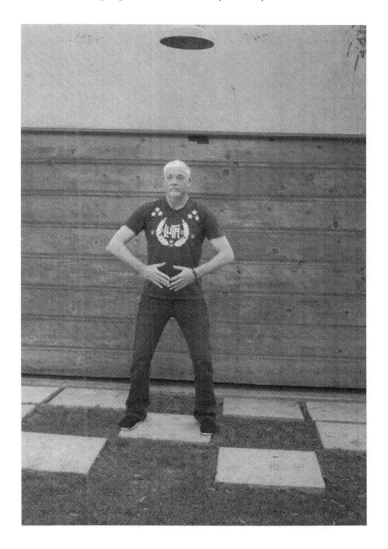

ENTER THIS URL TO WATCH THE DEMO VIDEO
"Building the Qi":
https://youtu.be/UWqB1dJn4ZM

7— EASY MOVEMENTS: SET 2

("Eagles Flight with the Sun and Moon" The Mood Enhancement Set)

This first set is a beautiful and enjoyable set of Qigong movements. Some T.C.M. doctors believe that these movements can bring about a natural mood enhancement. The movement's release a good amount of dopamine and are believed by some to counteract moodiness or "the blues."

EASY MOVEMENTS

We begin in the starting Qigong position

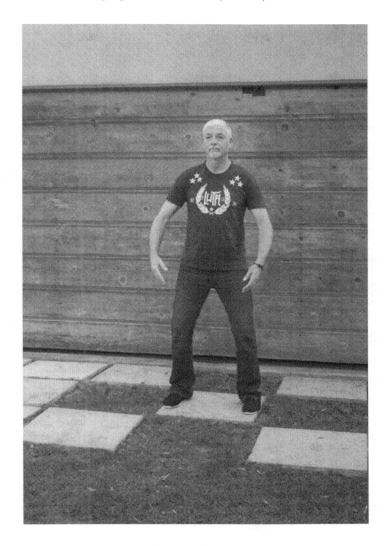

MOVEMENT #1: "Awakening the Qi"

We start this four movement form with the movement called, "Awakening the Qi."

The arms "float up" in front of us to a little below shoulder height. We inhale with our breath as we do this. Often there is a bit of a soft and fluid bend in the arms as we do this movement.

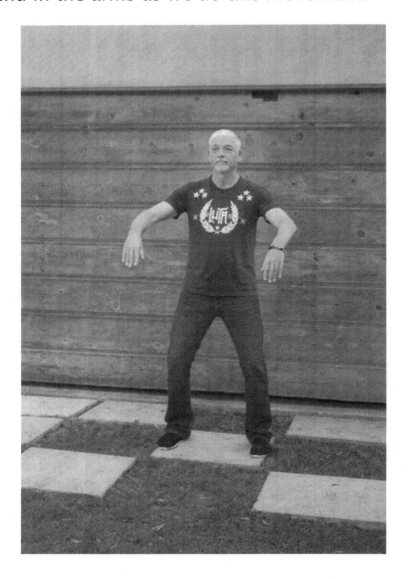

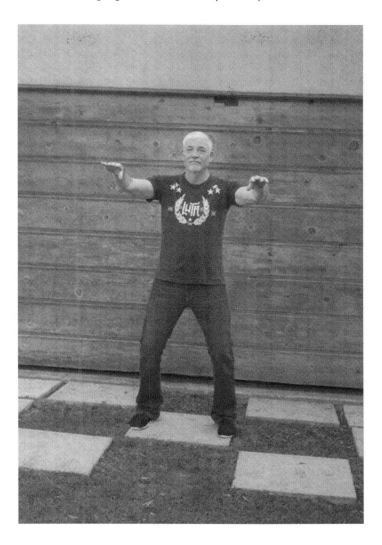

As we exhale, our arms float back down to the beginning position. We continue these arm movements in coordination with the inhalation and exhalation of our breath.

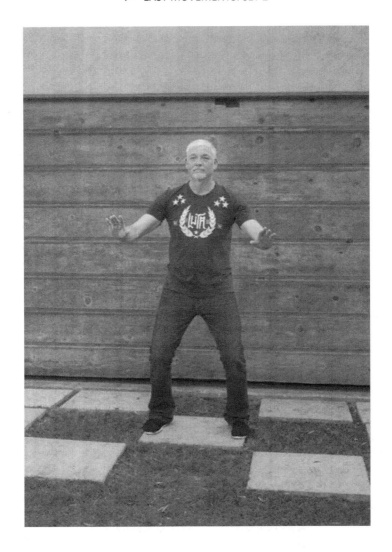

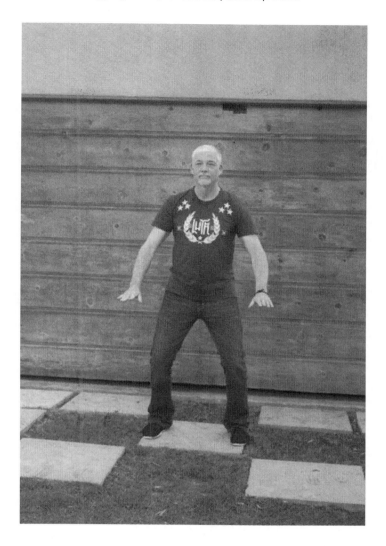

We can continue this for as many repetitions as we desire. If we do each of the movements approximately 10 times, the total time will be about 4 to 5 minutes.

When completed, return the beginning Qigong position, mentally check in on the "3 Intentful

Adjustments" (breath, posture, mental focus) as you pause to transition to Movement #2.

MOVEMENT #2: "Eagles Flight"

The second movement of the set is called, "Eagles Flight."

From the beginning Qigong position, we again have our arms "float up" from our sides, as if we were imitating an eagle moving its wings.

On the inhale, our arms ("wings") float up to about shoulder height. Again, there is a soft and fluid bend in our arms.

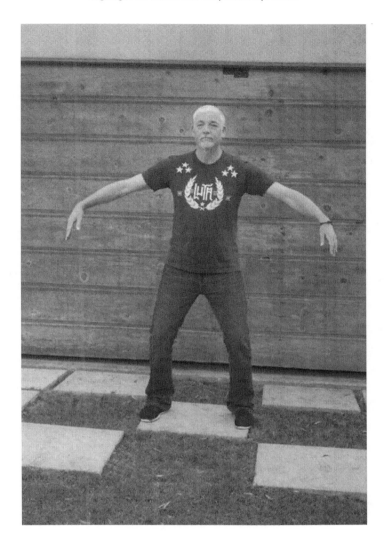

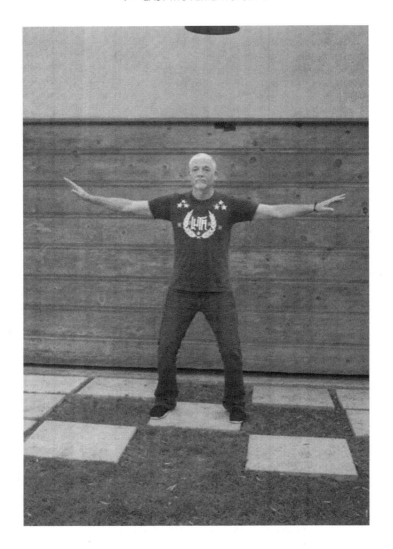

As we slowly exhale, our arms ("wings") gently float back down to our sides.

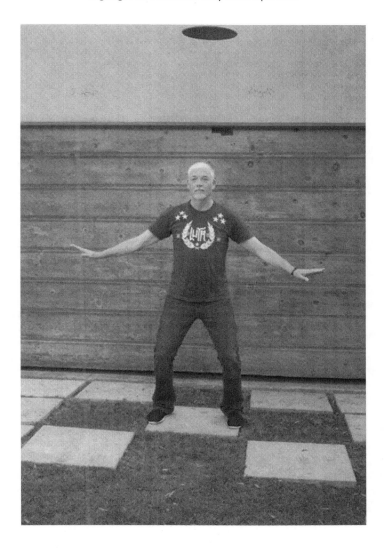

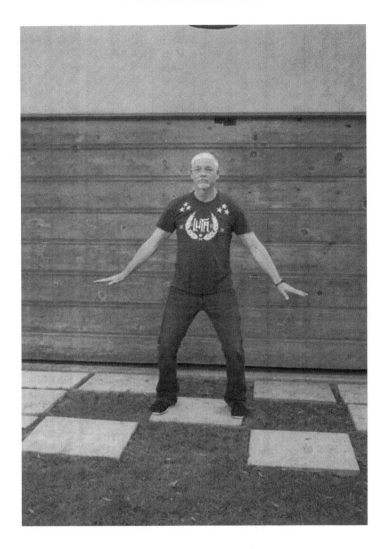

It is important to imagine that you are actually an eagle soaring high in the skies, while gently moving your wings. You may wish to close your eyes while doing this to assist your imagination in painting that picture for you as you do the movement.

Note that this movement can also be done as a "stand alone" movement that can be quickly done in order to calm oneself, center one self, or enhance your mood.

MOVEMENT #3: "Playing with the Sun"

The third movement of the set is called, "Playing with the Sun."

Once you transition from "Eagles Flight" back to the beginning position, you should begin to imagine you are a small child who is happy and playing with a ball. The "ball" you are playing with is the sun. It is important to smile as you do these movements, as if you are a carefree child lost in playing with a ball. Remember, imagination is the key to effective Qigong.

From the beginning Qigong position, slightly shift your weight onto your left leg, as you slowly move your right arm from your right side up to the left above your head, as if you were holding a ball and lifting it to toss it to the left. The palm of your hand is facing up, as if you were holding a basketball.

As you do this, your right foot raises to the toes and ball of the right foot (as if you wanted to reach higher), and the right heel of the foot lifts from the ground. This is in coordination with an inhale of your breath. Imagine you are slowly tossing a large ball to your left.

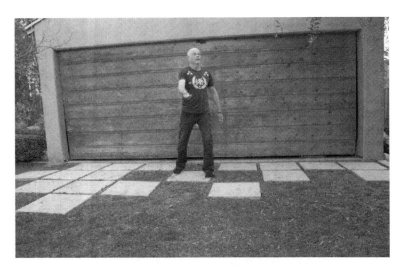

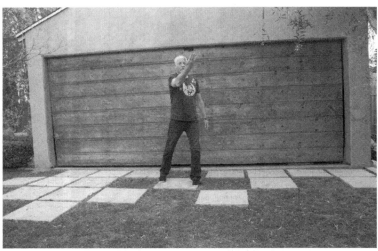

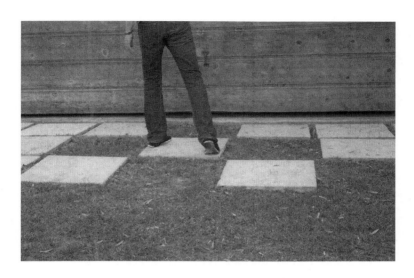

As you start to exhale, settle the weight again evenly between both legs, as you draw your hand back from the left to your right side.

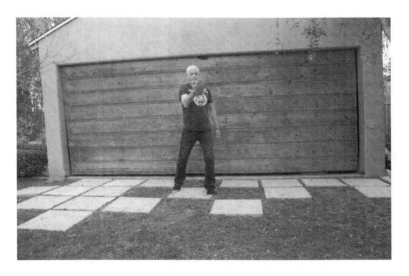

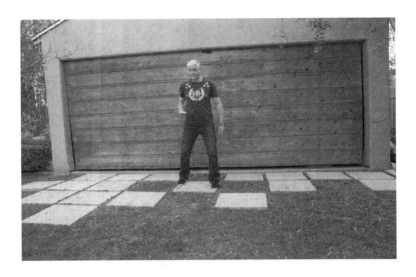

Now, repeat the movement with your left hand lifting "a ball" from your left side to your right, as your hand lift into the sky above your head and shoulders on the right.

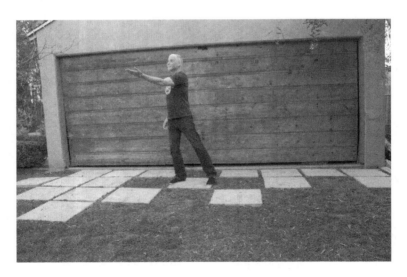

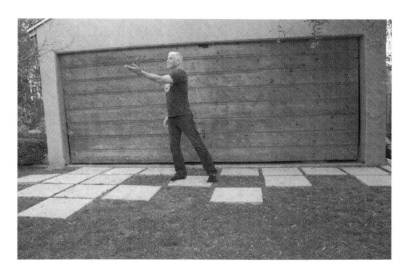

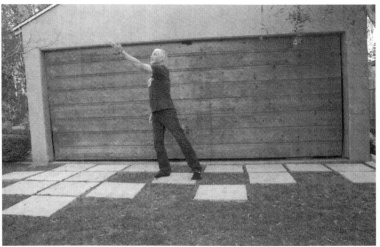

On the exhale, slowly draw the hand back as you let your left heel return to the ground and evenly distribute your weight again to both legs.

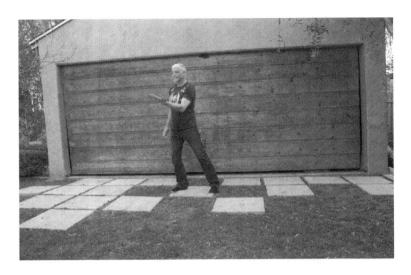

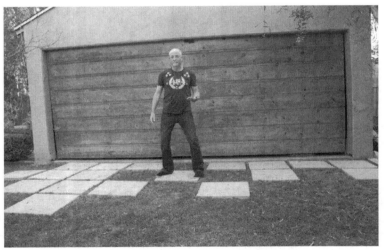

Repeat these movements to the right and to the left for as many repetitions as your desire.

Remember to imagine you are a child playing with the sun as if it were a ball, a smile on your face, and a carefree attitude. This will enhance the release of the dopamine into your system.

Upon completion, return to the beginning Qigong position.

MOVEMENT #4: "Gazing at the Moon"

The fourth movement is called, "Gazing at the Moon."

From the beginning Qigong position, gently lift both hands (palm up) to about chest level and turn towards your back, looking at your hands as they gently lift above your shoulders to the rear. Here, you hold it for a second as you "gaze at the moon." Generally, this movement backwards is done as you slowly inhale. You exhale as your hands return to the front.

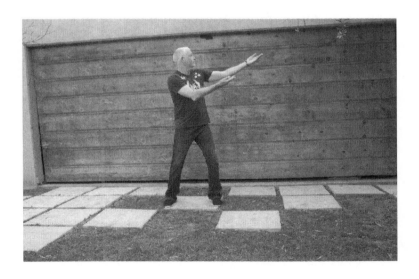

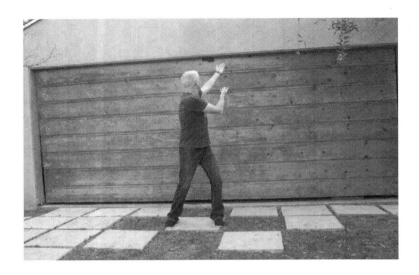

Slowly and gently, return your hands to the front of your chest.

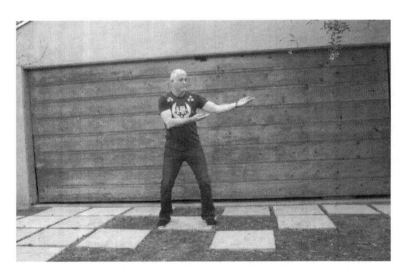

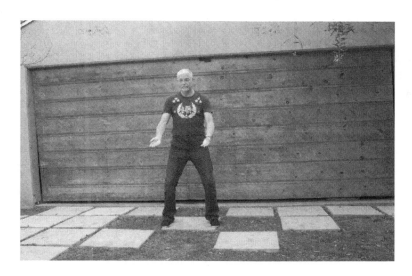

Do the same thing on the other side in a continuous motion.

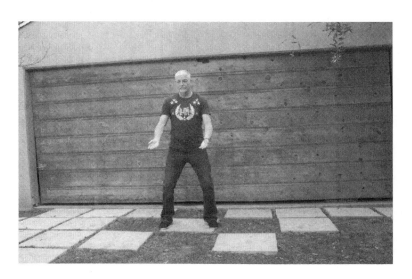

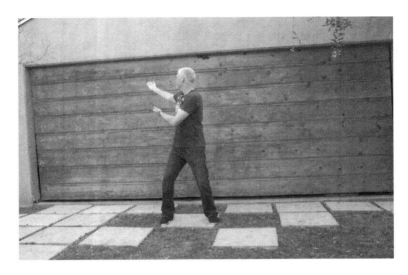

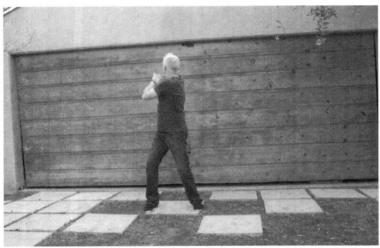

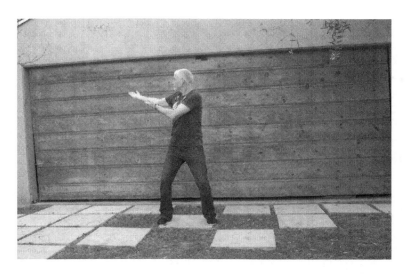

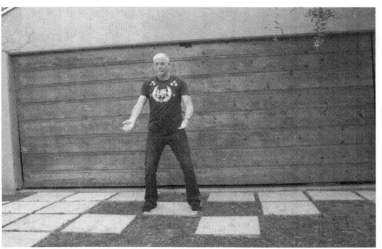

Keep your spine straight and upright as you turn in all these movements. Though it is a wonderful stretch for your back, neck, and spine, but *do not force the stretch too much.* Only stretch to about 75 % capacity and stay within your own comfort zone. Over time your flexibility will improve.

Continue this for as many repetitions as you desire. Again, if you do each one of these movements approximately 10 times each, the total time of this Qigong set will add up on the average to about 4 to 5 minutes.

This particular movement is excellent for stretching the back and keeping the spinal system limber. Since many people spend their work day sitting in a chair and looking at a computer, it is extremely helpful to do exercises that stretch and elongate the spinal column.

Once you are done with this movement, you can return to the beginning Qigong position and prepare for the closing.

CLOSING: "Sealing the Qi"

The closing movement is called, "Sealing the Qi."

From the beginning Qigong position, you move your hands out in front on your lower abdomen ("Dan Tien") and inhale as you "scoop up" the 'Qi/oxygen.' Your hands and arms will be slightly curved and horizontal in front of your lower abdomen.

As you exhale, push the Qi in towards your belly button.

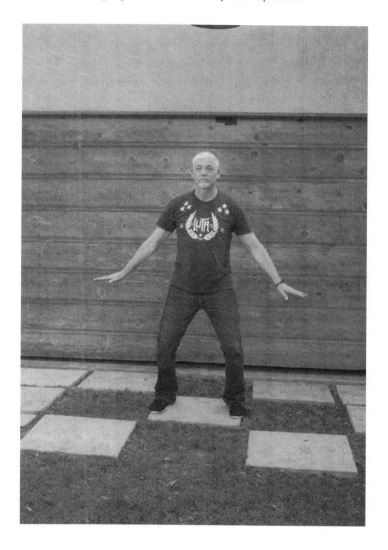

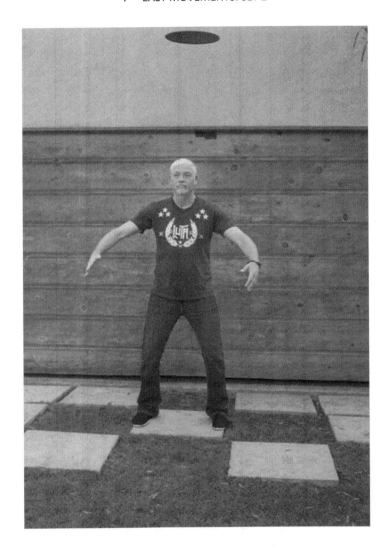

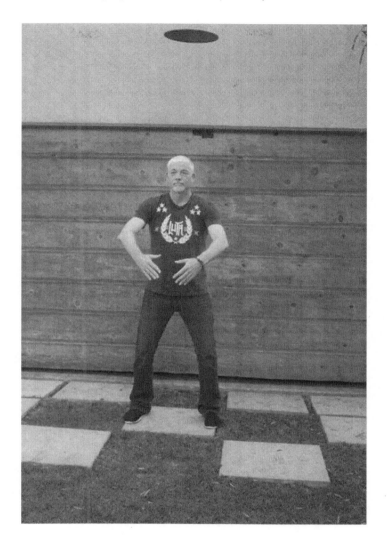

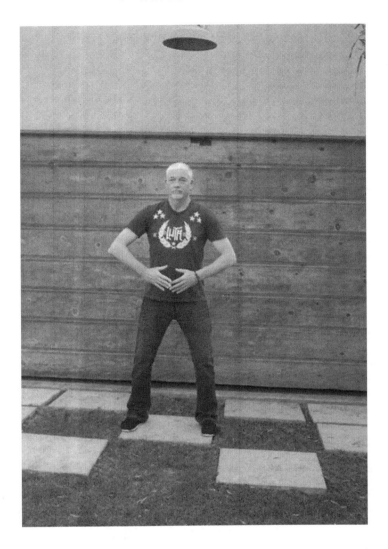

Repeat this movement three times in order to "seal your Qi" with this closing movement.

ENTER THIS URL TO WATCH THE DEMO VIDEO:
"Eagles Flight With the Sun and Moon"
https://youtu.be/PlPU1nVlkMM

8 – EASY MOVEMENTS: SET 3

("Immunity Booster Set")

This set of Qigong movements is called the "Immunity Booster Set." If you begin to feel a tickle in your throat, fatigue, or a runny nose, etc., then it is time to integrate these movements into your regular Qigong practice. These movements come from a very common Medical Qigong form called, "Medical Vitality Method."

EASY MOVEMENTS

MOVEMENT #1: "Awakening the Qi"

We start this four movement form with the movement called, "Awakening the Qi."

The arms "float up" in front of us to a little below shoulder height. We inhale with our breath as we do this. Often there is a bit of a soft and fluid bend in the arms as we do this movement.

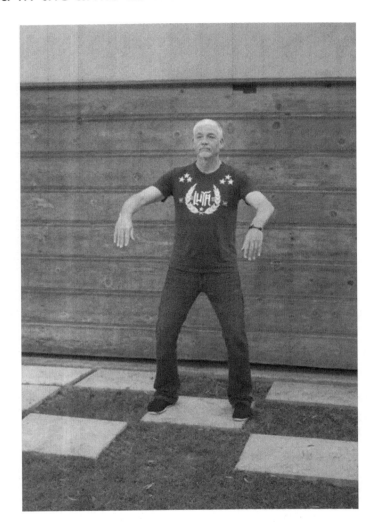

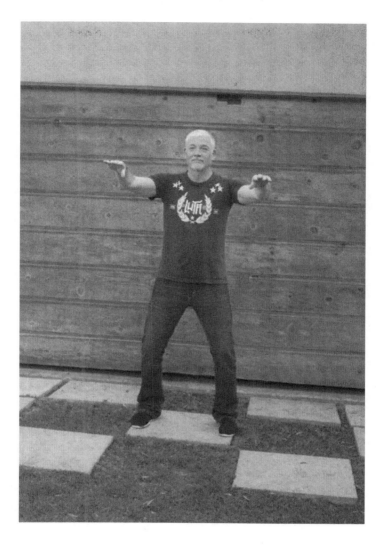

As we exhale, our arms float back down to the beginning position.

We continue these arm movements in coordination with the inhalation and exhalation of our breath.

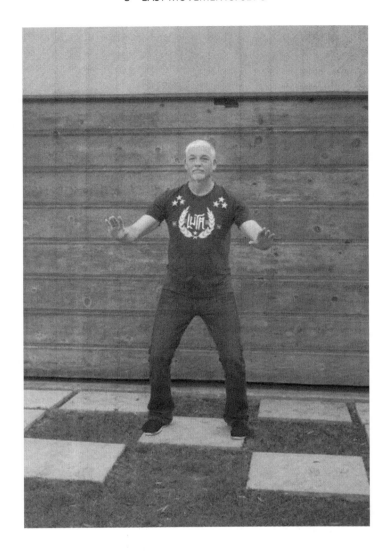

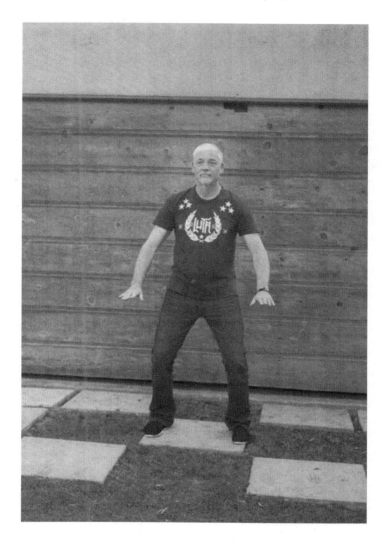

MOVEMENT #2: "Pushing the World Off of Your Shoulders"

This movement is a bit unusual among Qigong movements, in that there is *some* contraction of the muscles, not unlike Isometric exercises. As you do the individual movements of this exercise, you need to imagine you are pushing heavy objects with your whole body and your arms, and engage your muscles accordingly.

For example, the first part of the movement involves your palms lifting up from shoulder height, and imagining you are pushing a heavy globe off of your shoulders. Think of "Atlas" lifting the globe above his shoulders. This movement is done slowly as if lifting a genuine heavily weighted object. Once your arms are fully extended, you soften and relax the muscles of the arms and shoulders and bring them back to the center beginning position.

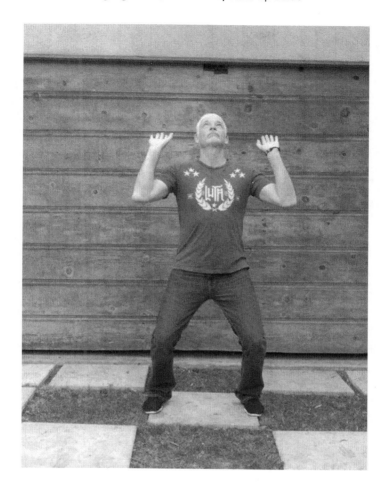

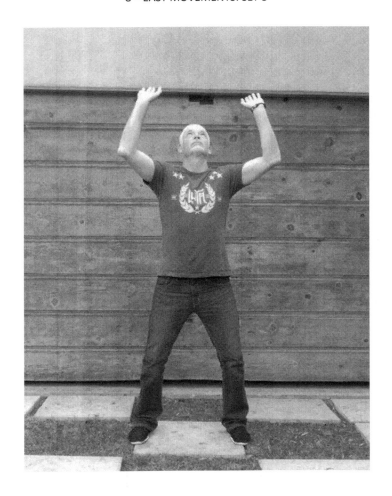

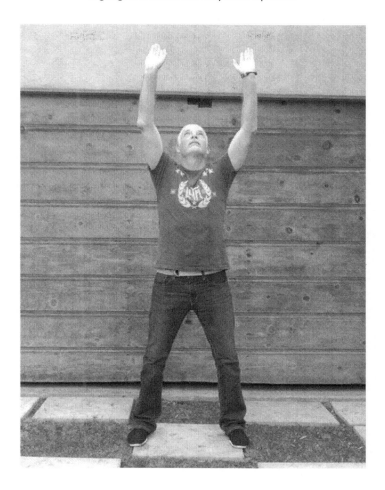

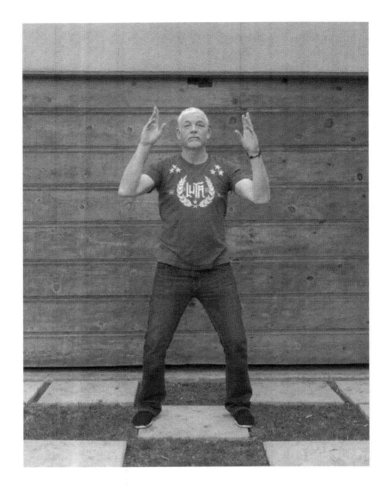

The second part of this movement involves pushing straight in front of you, as if you were pushing a car that had stalled. Your arms, shoulders and muscles engage as you slowly push forward in front of you. Once the arms are fully extended, the muscles again soften and relax, then draw back towards the center.

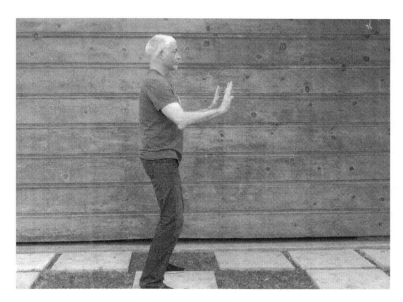

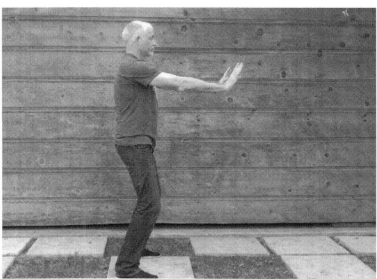

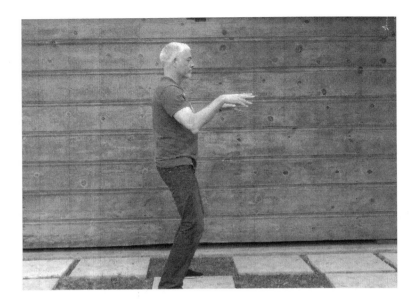

For the third movement, imagine you are pushing away walls that are pushing in on you. (Remember the scene from the first "Star Wars" film when the heroes are stuck in the trash compactor, pushing the walls back that are crushing in on them?).

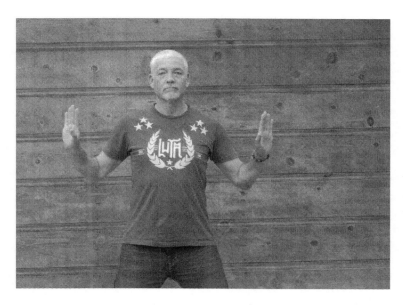

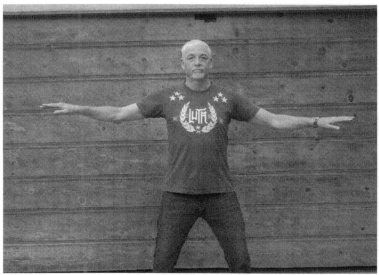

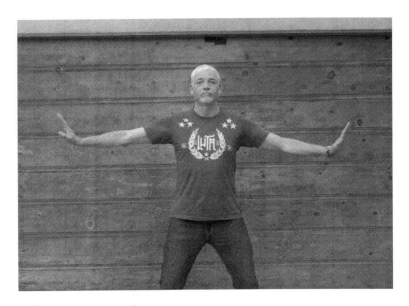

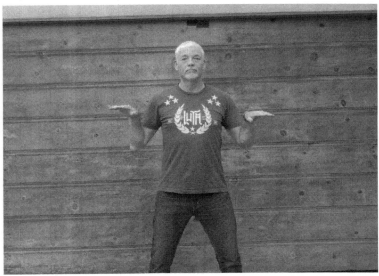

For the fourth portion of the exercise, entails placing the palms of your hands at waist level, then pushing down very strongly as if you were lifting your body out of the edge of a pool. Once the arms are fully extended, they softly disengage, relax, and return to center.

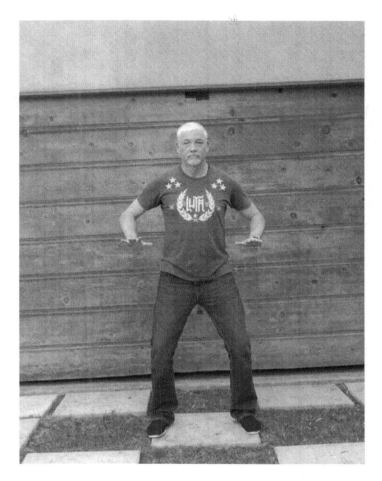

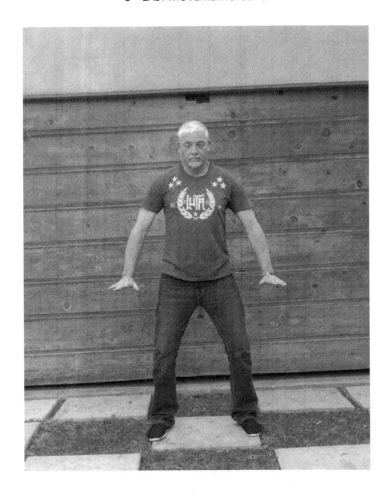

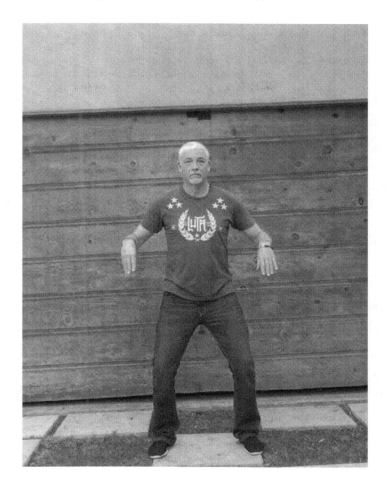

To review, the first movement engages the shoulders and the arms in pushing the heavy world off of your shoulders. The second movement engages the whole torso, shoulders and arms, pushing hard against an obstacle in front of you. Imagine you are pushing a stalled car. The third movement, you imagine you are pushing away walls that are crushing in on you. The fourth and final portion of the movement engages the arms in pushing from the waist slowly downwards, as if we are lifting our body out of the side of a pool.

Each of these four movements are repeated for three sets. Some people find it helpful when they are pushing to exhale their breath slowly and audibly. This adds intensity and focus to the movement. Once the arms are completely extended, remember to completely relax the arms and shoulders as you inhale and draw the hands back to center.

To enhance the exercise, imagine that *symbolically*, as you "lift the world off your shoulders," you are doing so with your worries, cares, and troubles. As "you push the car in front of you," imagine you are moving a major obstacle to your success and happiness out of the way. On the third movement, when you are "pushing back on enclosing walls," imagine you are freeing yourself of stifling constraints. On the forth movement, as you "lift your body out of the pool," imagine you are lifting yourself out of the complications and struggles of the world, and getting to a place of freedom. These may seem like silly thoughts, but connecting physical movements with emotionally releasing and healing thoughts is a very powerful combination.

Some people find this particular movement, "Lifting the World Off of Your Shoulders," To be helpful in releasing blockages of energy.

MOVEMENT #3: "Kidney Circles"

Stand in the beginning Qigong position and make your hands into fists. Not tight fists, but just simply ball them up, and keep them closed. Move your hands to your back immediately over the kidneys. Begin doing small circles. When it is colder during the wintertime, move the circles *in* towards the spine. During the warm summer months, move the direction of the circles outward away from the body. Do whatever number of repetitions feels comfortable to you. Chinese tradition states, "If you do 1000 kidney circles each day, then you will live for 1000 years." Some teachers' recommend you do at least as many circles as the number of years of your age. T.C.M. considers the kidneys one of the key organ systems that determine our health. This exercise is considered extremely important in T.C.M. in order to maintain and improve one's health.

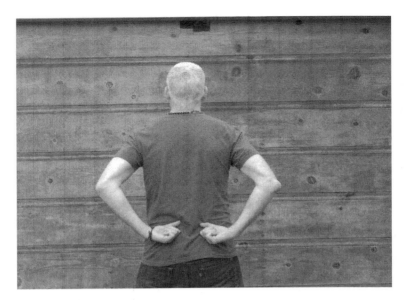

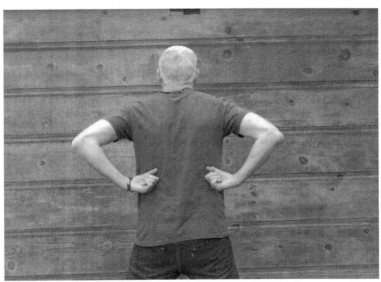

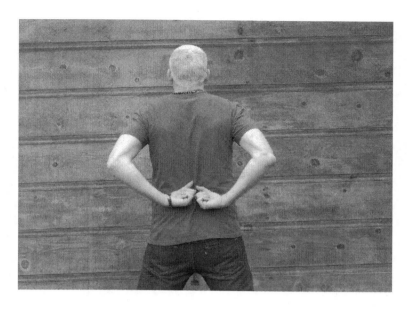

MOVEMENT #4: "Tracing the Meridian Channels."

Come back to the beginning Qigong position. Place the palm of your hands on the kidneys. Gently stroke your palms down past your buttocks, to the back of the legs, down the calves, then circle around the sides of your feet (It helps to bend your knees a little to be able to reach down). Continue lightly stroking your palms up of the "inside" of your calves, thighs, up the pelvic area, stomach, center of the chest, up the neck, until the fingers are pressing up near your ears and hairline (Hold for a second or two, for the "free facelift"). Then, continue pressing the fingers up the center of the skull, down the back, then trace your fingers around in a circle just above your ears (like the top of a pumpkin being cut off), Then, come back around the middle of the forehead, center of the skull, and trace down the back of the neck muscles, over the top of your shoulders, past your collarbone to the center of your chest. Then move your palms along your ribs as they slide over to your back and kidneys, Then we begin the motion all over again. The breathing is deep, even, and relaxed. The movement is slow, and the pressure on the skin is extremely light.

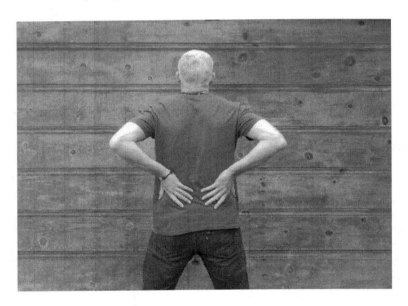

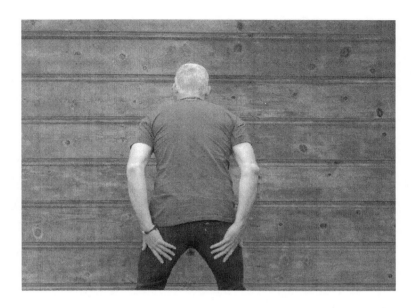

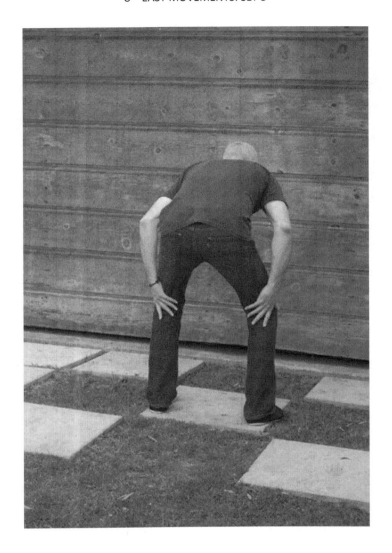

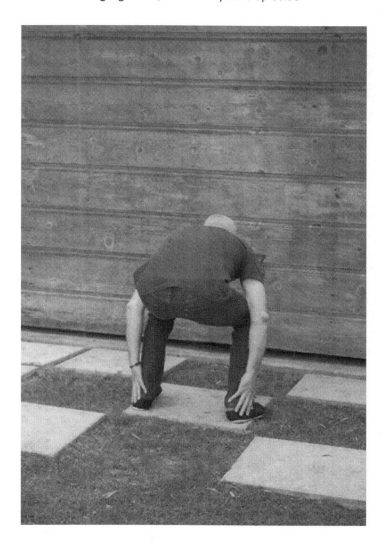

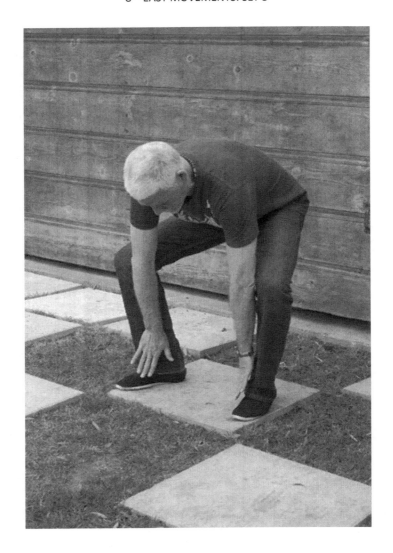

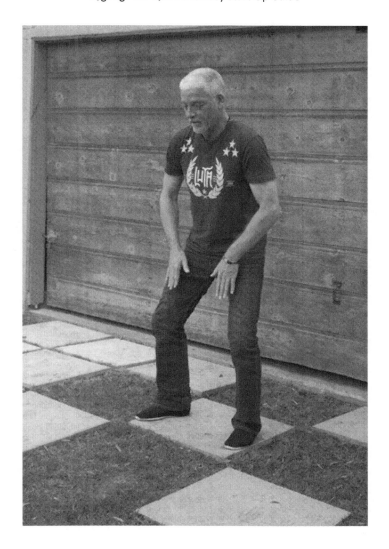

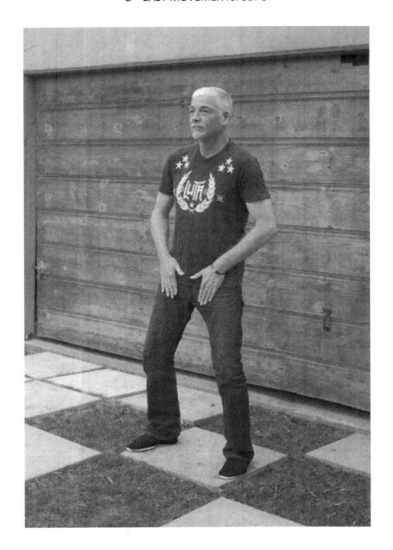

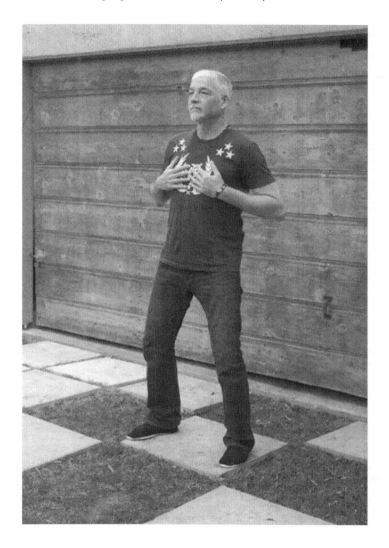

After approximately 5 to 10 repetitions of that movement, when your hands return to the center of the chest, begin stroking the outside of your outstretched arm from the hand, up to the shoulder, upper side of the neck, over the top of the head, onto the other side the head, then down your sternum through the groin area. Now, the other hand traces the outside of the other arm in the same way. Once the outside of the arms have been stroked, the palms gently stroke the inside of the arm, up the shoulder, up the neck, over the ears, down the other side of the head, then down the sternum through to the groin area. Now repeat with the other hand on the inside part of the other arm. Do this repetition another 4 to 6 times.

To conclude this movement, complete another 3 to 6 repetitions of the first movement (tracing the torso and legs). Return to the beginning Qigong position.

MOVEMENT #5: CLOSING: "Sealing the Qi"

The closing movement is called, "Sealing the Qi."

From the beginning Qigong position, you move your hands out in front on your lower abdomen ("Dan Tien") and inhale as you "scoop up" the 'Qi/Oxygen.' Your hands and arms will be slightly curved and horizontal in front of your lower abdomen.

As you exhale, push the Qi in towards your belly button.

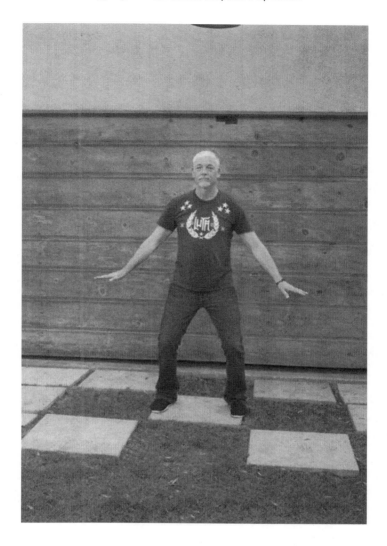

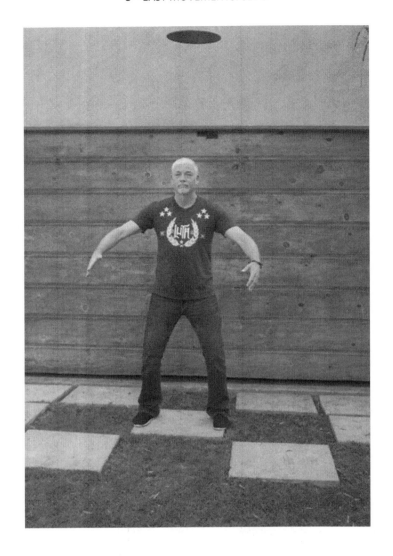

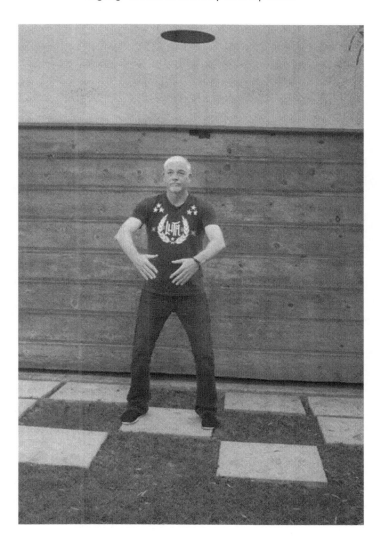

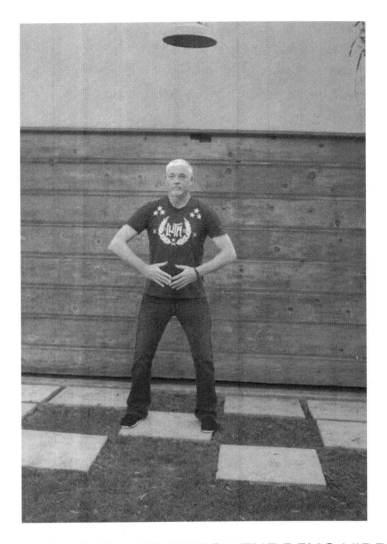

ENTER THIS URL TO WATCH THE DEMO VIDEO:
"Immunity Booster Set"
https://youtu.be/0ZZk7glWmuY

9 – EASY MOVEMENTS: SET 4

("Cleansing Organs with Light")

This particular set of Qigong exercises is extremely easy to do on a physical level, since it is a standing Qigong and no movement is involved. But in some ways, it is an "advanced set," because it involves more focus, concentration, and imagination of the mind.

EASY MOVEMENTS

The "Cleansing Organs with Light" set begins and ends in the basic beginning Qigong position. Rather than have your hands at your sides and away from your body, you can also move your palms In front of your lower abdomen approximately 6 to 12 inches away from the skin. Point the palms towards the "Dan Tien."

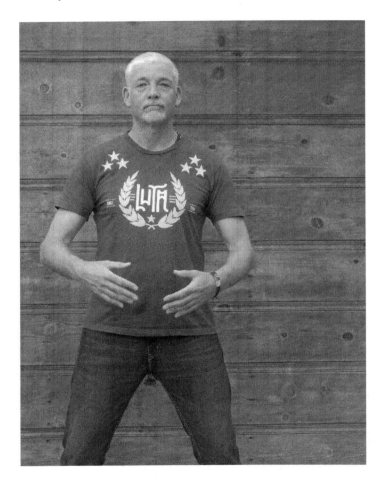

Take a few minutes to close your eyes and do a quick head to toe body relaxation. Now the real work begins. This is where we will call upon the power of the mind and the imagination. Our body believes whatever we tell it. The "Cleansing Organs with Light" set rests upon your power of visualization within your own mind.

With your eyes closed as your body stands in the beginning Qigong position, draw your mental attention to your lungs. As you inhale, draw a beautiful and vibrant white light into the lungs. As you exhale, breathe out a dirty greyish-white light (imagine the pure white light being polluted with smog). Inhale the bright and beautiful white light into your lungs five times. Exhale the dirty polluted greyish-white light five times as you exhale, imagine all the toxins that has accumulated in your lungs being expelled and released from your body into the air.

With your eyes continuing to stay closed, move your minds focus on to your kidneys. Inhale a clean, strong, pitch-black onyx light into the kidneys with each breath, As you exhale, imagine the black light again being polluted with a dull, dusty, muddled softer black color. Imagine the shiny deep, dark, obsidian -onyx light that you breathe into your kidneys is cleansing and renewing their core strength. The polluted, muddled, mixed with dirty-grey light that you exhale removing all of the toxins that have accumulated in your kidneys. We inhale the rich clean and beautiful black onyx light five times. We exhale the dirty, dull, muddled, grayish-black light five times.

Next we move our minds-eye to our liver we imagine a rich emerald forest green light filling our liver on each inhalation. As we exhale the toxins from our liver, we imagine a dull, greenish-gray, dirty light being expelled from our liver, into our breath, and out of our body. We inhale the chloroform emerald green healing light into our liver five times. We exhale the toxin-filled dirty, dull greenish- gray light from our liver through our breath, and then out into the air five times.

Now we bring our attention to our heart. As we inhale we imagine a beautiful deep red, bright healing light coming into the four chambers of our heart. As we exhale, a weak, dull, reddish-pink light with white small lumps in it is expelled into the air. With each inhalation, a rich ruby-red cleansing light expands the chambers of the heart and loosens any clogging and deposits of cholesterol. As we exhale we breathe out these deposits of toxins. We inhale the rich red cleansing light five times. We exhale the dirty, pale, polluted red light five times.

The last organ system we focus our attention on is the spleen. As we inhale, we imagine a beautiful bright yellow light energetically flowing into our spleen. With each inhalation as we exhale, we breathe out a dull greenish-yellow light and expel the accumulated toxins into the air. We breathe in the bright daisy-yellow light five times. We exhale the toxin laden, dull greenish-yellow light five times.

We finish the "Cleansing Organs with Light" set by imagining a bright healing warm white light filling our entire body with each inhalation. With each exhalation the same vibrant white light is released into the air. We have bathed our organs in healing light so there are now no more toxins to expel. The light that we breathe in is clean and pure. The white light breath that we exhale is clean and pure. We do this final breath cycle five times. five installations, then five exhalations. Our body has been cleansed of toxins, and feels light, clean, and free.

10 – EASY MOVEMENTS: SET 5

("Wudang Standing Qigong)

For centuries the Daoist monks of Wudang Mountain have generated some of the deepest and most profound Qigong exercises to come out of China, the birthplace of Qigong. Though we may not have the opportunity to spend years of concerted Qigong and Martial Arts training like the monks, we can benefit from incorporating some of their exercises into our modern lifestyles. Below is just one of the profound Wudang Standing Qigong exercises that can enhance our health and wellbeing.

EASY MOVEMENTS

MOVEMENT #1: "Standing Qigong"

We begin this set with the beginning Qigong position, with the palms of the hands facing our lower abdomen / "Dan Tien" area. Stand comfortable with eyes closed. Do not try to imagine or focus on anything. Simply relax into the position and breathe diaphragmatically and deeply. Let calmness center you. If your mind wanders or you get distracted, simply listen to and feel your breath. Maintain this position for a few minutes.

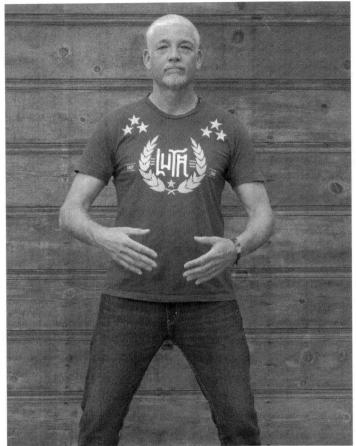

Movement #1: Standing Qigong

Movement #2: "Wudang Flowing Motion"

Open your eyes about halfway, keeping the muscles around the eyes soft. Slowly move your hands so the finger tips face one another, palm up, just a little apart. With an inhale move your hands and palms up in unison up along the left side of your body, from the top of your thigh, up the left side of the torso, to about shoulder height. As you begin to exhale, turn the palms over and flow down along the same pathway. Once at the bottom, turn palms up again and inhale moving along the same path. Repeat this pattern about 4 times. On the fifth pass up as the hands reach shoulder length, turn the palms over and repeat the same movements to the right side. Alternate sides after about four or so complete passes. Do this a few times. Do not get too serious about the number of times you do the movements on each side, just try to make sure they are done an even number (approximately) on each side.

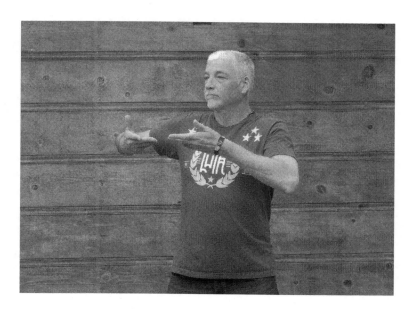

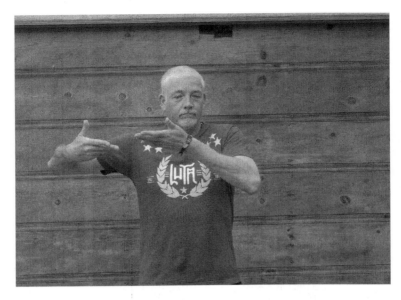

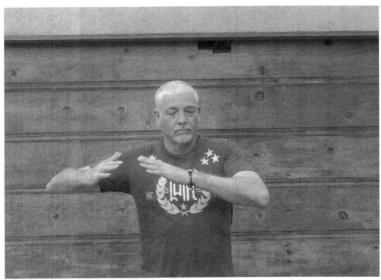

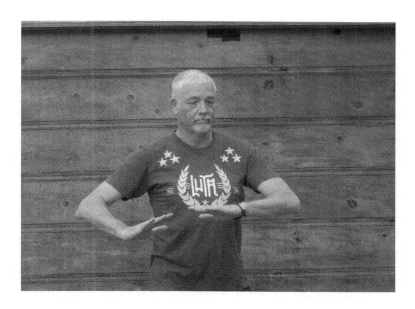

CLOSING: "Sealing the Qi"

The closing movement is called, "Sealing the Qi."

From the beginning Qigong position, you move your hands out in front on your lower abdomen ("Dan Tien") and inhale as you "scoop up'' the 'Qi/Oxygen.' Your hands and arms will be slightly curved and horizontal in front of your lower abdomen.

As you exhale, push the Qi in towards your belly button.

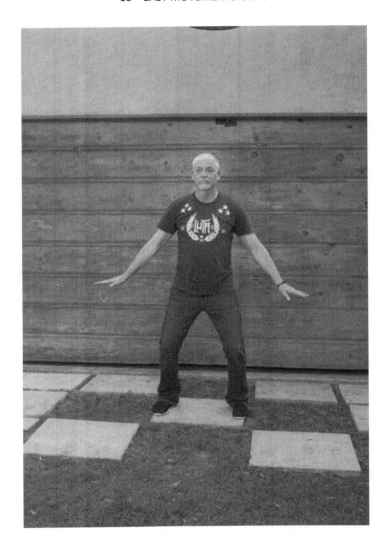

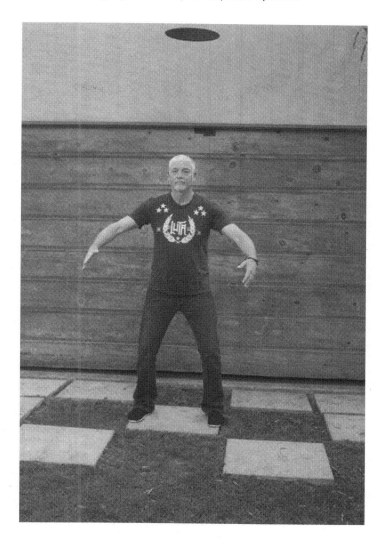

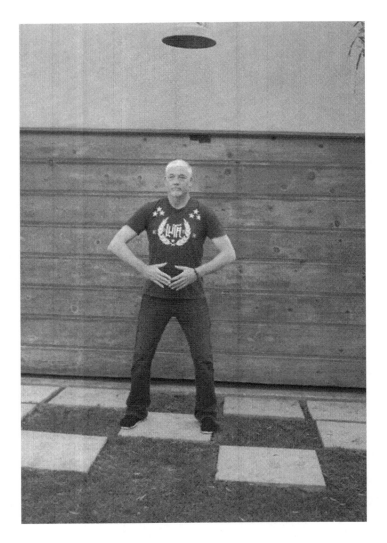

ENTER THIS URL TO WATCH THE DEMO VIDEO:
"Wudang Standing Qigong"
https://youtu.be/RPGLkAzIf60

11 – EASY MOVEMENTS: SET 6

("Wudang Sleeping Qigong")

There is a long tradition within ancient Daoist circles of developing Qigong exercises to use when one is preparing to sleep, or simply lying down. For those who are reluctant to exercise, or to attempt learning mind/body practices, this Qigong exercise is about the easiest any exercise can get, since you do it lying down!

This particular supine Qigong comes from the Daoist tradition of Wudang Mountain. It is good overall Qi building and preserving movement. The idea is that as you prepare to sleep for the evening, you would move into this position, and concentrate on breathing in the Qi into your lower abdomen ("Dan Tien")

MOVEMENT #1:

Lie down on your right side. Open the fingers and thumbs of both hands wide, but without straining them (This is called "Tiger Hands"). Place your right "Tiger Hand" along your cheekbone and ear on the right side of your head and rest it on the hand (you can also have the hand and head propped on a thin pillow underneath).

Pull the knees of both legs close to your abdomen (somewhat like in a fetal position). Place the left knee resting on the right knee. Gently place the left heel of your foot onto the top part of your right calf. Then take your right "Tiger Hand" and rest it on your lower abdomen ("Dan Tien"). Close your eyes, relax, and imagine the thin stream of your breath/Qi coming through the top of your head ("Bai Hui") down into your "Dan Tien" area.

For as long as you are conscious, maintain this visualization, but let your mind drift asleep naturally. If you awaken in the night as you sleep, you can continue the visualization if you wish.

If you grow stiff in this position, or simply want to turn over, you can do the same position and visualization on your left side as well; simply reverse all the movements and positions to the other side.

How many mind/body systems encourage you to perform the "exercises" as you sleep, or are lying down? As I mentioned in the introduction, in Mainland China, hospital patients who are bed-ridden are sometimes prescribed specific Qigong forms to do while in a supine position. The ancient practice of Qigong takes all of our lifestyles and conditions as human beings into account. It seeks to flow with the natural order of how humans live and respect the ebbs and flows of our daily lives. Qigong is Ancient Philosophical Daoism 101 in practice.

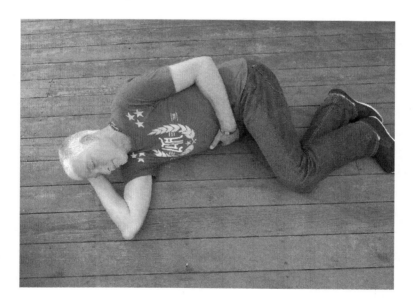

NON-CONCLUSION

I named this chapter "non"-conclusion to emphasize a very important point. There is no "conclusion" or final arrival point in the path of Qigong. I do not mean this in some esoteric or mystical sense. Qigong is a rich resource and the treasures that can be drawn from it are endless. Qigong is a path that never ends, so how can it "conclude?" As you grow to enjoy the sensations, peace, calm, and health benefits that come from doing Qigong, you will want to do it more. You will want to get into deeper, and internalize the principles so that the benefits are yours all the time, not just when you are doing Qigong.

Stepping onto this path of Qigong can open many other roads in life that you never would have dreamed of. Over time, you may begin to develop a better sense of intuition, which is a powerful tool for life-success. Your artistic and creative, or your analytical and concentration skills may improve (Doing movements from the left to the right over a period of time can balance the "right-brain/left-brain" patterns within your brain). Things previously difficult will become easier. Perceptions and insights that you never would have seen before open up as you become more relaxed, centered, and focused. All of these benefits have occurred in my life without some extraordinary investment of time and effort on my part. I simply love to do Qigong on a regular basis for a few minutes a day (I usually do at least 20 minutes, some days 40 minutes, at the most).

Just doing 10 minutes a day for a few years caused the positive changes mentioned above to occur in my life. What I love most about Qigong is that you get back what you invest into it *many times over*. The "R.O.I." (Return on Investment) is exponential. In many aspects of life, you get back what you put into it; "you reap what you sow." Investing in Qigong practice is like "sowing" into fertilized, composted, high yield garden soil. Drop in the seeds, throw a little water on it, and in a short amount of time you reap a bountiful harvest of enhanced health, stress reduction, and mental focus.

Like anything, the more you invest in Qigong the more benefits you will receive. If you do Qigong, but also smoke a pack of cigarettes, drink a 12-pack of beer, and eat fast food each day, your benefits will not be as great as someone who does not make those choices. But ironically, making a small commitment to do Qigong for a few minutes a day can help you make those other changes in your life you know you should. The focus and peace that comes from Qigong can help in breaking the hold of unhealthy addictions. Many addiction centers and therapists are beginning to use Qigong as a modality in their work with clients.

Qigong can help open a door to many positive changes in your life. The key is to not put too much pressure on yourself, and end up turning it into "work." You may need some level of self-discipline to be consistent with regular Qigong practice. But do not beat yourself into the ground if you only do it 4 days a week instead of 7, or for 7 minutes a day instead of 20 minutes a day. Do not be in a hurry to "master" Qigong. Simply be as consistent as possible, have fun, enjoy the sacredness of time spent for yourself and your health. Then you will not need to master Qigong, it will master you. The benefits will build up in your life just as surely as the sun rises every day without you having to help bring it up. Be committed to yourself, treasure yourself, and the blessings of Qigong practice will flow into your life in due time.

In future publications, I will explore some of the many applications that Qigong has in areas like sports, business, romance, creative efforts, and many other realms of the human experience. To unpack the hosts of benefits can take a lifetime. All of these resources are available simply by integrating these simple and organic ancient time-tested health practices into your daily life.

Congratulations on beginning this positive change in your life. Enjoy the sacred silence, peace, and calm of Qigong. Your Qigong practice will provide an oasis of rest from our stressful world. Let no one deprive you of this time. It is a precious gift we can freely give to ourselves each new day. Our difficult and stressful times demand we be strong and calm. Let the power of Qigong be one of your sources of strength for daily living. The blessings of walking this path will abound to you and those you care for.

QIGONG CLASS HANDOUT

GENERAL GUIDELINES FOR QIGONG EXERCISE MOVEMENTS

PRINCIPLES OF THE "THREE INTENTFUL ADJUSTMENTS."
by
Frank Blaney

The "3 Intentful Adjustments" in relation to Qigong and Tai Chi movements are our *posture*, *breathing*, and *mental focus*.

POSTURE & BODY POSITION

--The top of the head (the crown or in Chinese, the "Bai Hui") is suspended as if by a string from heaven. This elongates the spinal column and tends to tilt the chin down a bit. The neck remains straight, but relaxed, not tensed.

--Arms do not lift up; instead think of the elbows "floating" up and outward, away from the torso. This will leave a small ball of air in the armpit area, approximately the size of an egg.

--Wrists are soft, slightly bent, hands and fingers are relaxed.

--Shoulders are soft, relaxed, and rounded. Imagine they are like warm oil slipping off the top of the torso.

--The lower back should straighten out, as if flat against a wall. This is done by *slightly* tilting the pelvis forward. Imagine your pelvis is a metal bowl with milk in it and unless you "level it out" the milk will spill. DO NOT OVEREXTEND THE PELVIS, AS THIS MAY CAUSE UNNECCESSARY STRAIN ON THE LOWER BACK! Follow the adage, "less is more." On the average, the shift is only a ½ inch to an inch. Find your own perfect position slowly over time as you stay in your comfort zone.

--Knees are slightly bent and never extend past the foot during any movements (this can overextend the tendons of the knees.)

--Imagine the bottom of your feet have literal "roots" that run down deep into the ground about eight feet. This will aid in your balance.

--All movements are slow, soft, and tend to move in an orbit or in circles. It is believed that the "Qi," (or "Ki" in Japanese) tends to move more powerfully in circular or orbital patterns throughout the body.

--Periodically "check in" on your posture and relaxation. Pay particular attention to the areas that tend to hold tension (the abdominal area, pelvis, neck, shoulders, eyes, head and face muscles). Purposefully *relax* these both before and during the Qigong exercise practices. Even Qigong "masters" still have to do this during their practice, so do not get frustrated while practicing because you are not constantly in "perfect" posture. No one is. In fact, some believe it is the contraction and expansion between our "perfect Qigong posture" and our regular "poor posture" that aids in the "pumping" of the Qi through the body.

--The arms, head, torso, hips, and legs should move together as a unit in a connected way.

--It helps to occasionally remind yourself that the head should lift, the tail bone descends, and the center (our heart, sternum, and diaphragm) should "open." Try to imagine these things happening simultaneously within the space of a few breaths, and then proceed with the Qigong movements you are doing.

--All movements should be done as slow as possible, as if they are being done *underwater*. Occasionally, check your "speed" to see if you can slow your movements down even more.

BREATH

--Breathe deeply, slowly, diaphragmatically. Think of a newborn baby. Watch their belly. Their belly raises and lowers more than their chest. They naturally and instinctively do "Qigong breathing." We are trying to relearn our natural and unstressed form of breathing.

--Let the breath deepen naturally. Do not try to force the breath to hold more than the lungs are naturally capable of. Over time your lung capacity and ability to breathe deeply and slowly will increase.

--Imagine your breath not only going into your abdomen, but even into your lower back area. As you progress in your visualization skills, imagine the breath coming in not only through the mouth, but also through the top of the head, and even through the pours of the skin. As you become more familiar with your Qigong movements, you will be able to relax more and visualize the breath going into the heels of your feet.

--Generally, breathe in and out through the nose.

--If you forget the prescribed or recommended pattern of the breathing for your particular Qigong exercise, do not worry about it. It is more important that your feel comfortable than to be worrying about keeping up with the "inhale here, exhale here..." pattern. Let your breath dictate the speed of your body movements, not vice versa.

--Feel free to experiment with what breathing patterns feel good to you. *Generally* (not always) movements that reach out tend to be exhales and movements that come in towards the torso tend to be inhales. This is true both in martial arts and Qigong.

--Notice that in your breathing pattern, the exhales tend to relax more, and the inhales tend to "nourish."

MENTAL FOCUS

--Do not try too hard to "get relaxed." Simply focus on the mundane things your body is doing, like the breathing pattern, or gazing at the movement of your hands during an exercise. One of the advantages of trying to get into a relaxed state with a moving meditation (vs. a still meditation) is that our mind is allowed to focus on *something* (like our breath or body movement) instead of some nebulous "inner peace" or "stillness" or "OOOMMMM," etc. Be "mindful" and "in the moment" simply by checking in with what your *body* is doing (the breath, the movements, the bodies' sensations, etc.).

--Do not get attached to feeling some sensation of Chi, euphoria, or whatever. If an exhilarating experience comes, experience it and let it go. Do not make these your goal. The benefits of Qigong are a lot like the other good habits of our life (eating right, exercising, taking your vitamins, getting adequate rest, etc.); you may not get an immediate "reward" or pleasurable sensation, but rather you will get beneficial long term rewards. Slow and steady wins the race. There is solid scientific proof that Qigong has tremendous health benefits. Do a little of it consistently and *you will* notice a positive difference over time.

--Try to cultivate an attitude of "cheerful indifference" during Qigong practice. Guard your mind against worrying about the past or future. Relish, savor, and drink deep of these minutes you have chosen to set aside for yourself and your health. Let the world and its concerns take care of itself while you take this precious time to replenish your storehouse of strength and spirit.

--As your Qigong movements become memorized and automatic, experiment with visualizing the breath extending throughout the body, both in the inhalations and exhalations. Some find this easier to do if they imagine the breath in colors; a cool blue for the pure air you inhale, a dirty brown or grey for the "dirty Chi" we exhale (imagine L.A. smog!). This mental visualization of the breath and Chi extending to the farthest reaches of our body actually helps *move* the Chi to these areas. This intensifies the tissue oxygenation, metabolic byproduct expulsion, and expands the immune systems healing properties to *all* the parts of our body.

ADDITIONAL RESOURCES

National Qigong Association

www.nqa.org

The Institute of Integral Qigong and Tai Chi

http://instituteofintegralqigongandtaichi.org/

Qigong Institute

www.qigonginstitute.org

The Healer Within Foundation

www.healerwithinfoundation.org

ABOUT THE AUTHOR

Frank Blaney was certified as a Qigong and Tai Chi Instructor in 2004 by the IIQTC (The Institute of Integral Qigong and Tai Chi), and has been practicing Qigong since 2000. Mr. Blaney is also a 2nd Degree Blackbelt in Budoshin Jujitsu, has studied various martial arts for many years, and has taught self-defense classes for women. He has a Bachelor's Degree with a focus on Intercultural Studies and a Master's Degree in Negotiation, Conflict Resolution, and Peace Building. He has worked for years as a violence prevention educator and social worker with at-risk youth in Los Angeles. He has served as the Chairperson for the Violence Prevention Coalition of Greater Los Angeles. Mr. Blaney is committed to sharing Qigong, Tai Chi, and holistic health practices with communities and organizations internationally. His vision is to empower individuals and communities with self-directed, sustainable, and low cost health-enhancement practices.

Made in the USA
Middletown, DE
29 May 2018